THE COMPLETE 2024 PROSTATE CANCER DIET COOKBOOK

105+ Tasty and Nutritional Friendly Recipes for Prostate Cancer Prevention and Recovery

LUCKY WILSON

Copyright © 2024 by Lucky Wilson

Table of Contents

INTRODUCTION

Introduction to Prostate Cancer and Nutrition

Understanding Prostate Cancer

Prostate cancer is one of the most common types of cancer affecting men, particularly those over the age of 50. The prostate is a small gland located below the bladder and in front of the rectum. It produces seminal fluid, which nourishes and transports sperm. Prostate cancer occurs when cells in the prostate gland begin to grow uncontrollably.

There are several risk factors associated with prostate cancer. Age is the most significant, with the majority of cases occurring in men over 65. Family history also plays a role; men with a father or brother who had prostate cancer are at increased risk. Additionally, genetic factors, race (with African American men being at higher risk), and lifestyle factors such as diet and exercise influence the likelihood of developing the disease.

Prostate cancer can be slow-growing or aggressive. Many men with prostate cancer do not experience symptoms in the early stages. However, as the disease progresses, symptoms may include difficulty urinating, blood in urine or semen, erectile dysfunction, and pain in the hips, back, or chest. Early detection through routine screening, such as prostate-specific antigen (PSA) tests and digital rectal exams (DRE), is crucial for effective treatment and management.

The Role of Diet in Prostate Cancer Prevention and Recovery

Nutrition plays a critical role in both the prevention and recovery from prostate cancer. A well-balanced diet can help reduce the risk of developing prostate cancer, slow its progression, and improve the quality of life for those undergoing treatment or in remission.

Research suggests that certain dietary patterns and foods are associated with a lower risk of prostate cancer. A diet rich in fruits, vegetables, whole grains, and lean proteins, with limited intake of red and processed meats, refined sugars, and high-fat dairy products, is beneficial.

Antioxidant-rich foods, such as tomatoes (high in lycopene), cruciferous vegetables (like broccoli and cauliflower), and berries, help protect cells from damage. Omega-3 fatty acids, found in fatty fish like salmon, as well as flaxseeds and walnuts, have anti-inflammatory properties that may help reduce cancer risk. Additionally, foods rich in vitamins D and E, selenium, and zinc are essential for maintaining prostate health.

Conversely, a diet high in saturated fats, trans fats, and excessive calorie intake is linked to an increased risk of prostate cancer. These dietary habits can lead to obesity, a known risk factor for various cancers, including prostate cancer. Therefore, maintaining a healthy weight through a balanced diet and regular physical activity is crucial.

For those already diagnosed with prostate cancer, nutrition can aid in managing side effects from treatments such as surgery, radiation, and hormone therapy. A nutrient-dense diet helps support the immune system, promotes healing, and maintains overall strength and energy levels. Specific dietary recommendations may vary depending on individual health needs and treatment plans, so consulting with a healthcare provider or a registered dietitian is advisable.

Overview of the Prostate Cancer Diet Cookbook

The Prostate Cancer Diet Cookbook is designed to provide a comprehensive guide to healthy eating for individuals seeking to prevent prostate cancer or support their recovery. This cookbook combines the latest nutritional research with delicious, easy-to-prepare recipes that cater to the dietary needs and preferences of those concerned about prostate health.

The cookbook is divided into several sections to make it user-friendly and accessible. The first section covers the basics of prostate cancer, including risk factors, symptoms, and the importance of early detection. It provides an overview of how diet and lifestyle choices can influence prostate health and reduce cancer risk.

The next section delves into the specifics of a prostate-healthy diet, highlighting key nutrients and food groups that have been shown to benefit prostate health. This includes detailed information on fruits, vegetables, lean proteins, whole grains, and healthy fats, along with tips on incorporating these foods into everyday meals.

The heart of the cookbook features a wide variety of recipes, ranging from breakfasts and snacks to main dishes and desserts. Each recipe is carefully crafted to be nutritious, flavorful, and easy to prepare. Nutritional information is provided for each recipe, helping readers make informed choices about their diet.

Additionally, the cookbook includes meal planning tips and sample meal plans to help users create balanced and satisfying menus. It also addresses common dietary challenges and provides practical solutions for maintaining a prostate-healthy diet while enjoying delicious food.

How to Use This Cookbook for Optimal Health

Using the Prostate Cancer Diet Cookbook effectively requires a commitment to adopting healthy eating habits and making informed food choices. Here are some tips to help you get the most out of this cookbook and support your prostate health:

1. Educate Yourself: Start by reading the introductory sections of the cookbook to gain a solid understanding of prostate cancer, its risk factors, and the role of diet in prevention and recovery. This knowledge will empower you to make better dietary decisions.

2. Plan Your Meals: Use the meal planning tips and sample meal plans provided in the cookbook to organize your

weekly meals. Planning ahead ensures you have the necessary ingredients on hand and reduces the likelihood of resorting to less healthy options.

3. Incorporate a Variety of Foods: Aim to include a wide range of fruits, vegetables, lean proteins, whole grains, and healthy fats in your diet. Variety not only ensures you get a broad spectrum of nutrients but also keeps meals interesting and enjoyable.

4. Focus on Portion Control: Pay attention to portion sizes to avoid overeating. The cookbook provides guidance on appropriate portion sizes for different types of foods, helping you maintain a healthy weight.

5. Experiment with Recipes: Try different recipes from the cookbook to discover new flavors and cooking techniques. Don't be afraid to modify recipes to suit your taste preferences or dietary restrictions.

6. Stay Hydrated: Drinking plenty of water is essential for overall health, including prostate health. The cookbook may include tips on incorporating hydrating foods and beverages into your diet.

7. Monitor Your Progress: Keep track of your dietary habits and how they make you feel. Regularly review your meal

plans and adjust them as needed to ensure you're meeting your nutritional needs and health goals.

8. Seek Professional Guidance: If you have specific dietary concerns or health conditions, consult with a healthcare provider or a registered dietitian. They can provide personalized advice and help you tailor the recipes and meal plans to your individual needs.

By following these guidelines and utilizing the Prostate Cancer Diet Cookbook, you can take proactive steps towards improving your prostate health and overall well-being. Remember, a healthy diet is a powerful tool in the fight against prostate cancer and can significantly enhance your quality of life.

Nutritional Guidelines for Prostate Cancer

Essential Nutrients for Prostate Health

Maintaining optimal prostate health and supporting recovery from prostate cancer involves focusing on several key nutrients known for their beneficial effects. Understanding these essential nutrients can help guide dietary choices that promote prostate wellness.

Lycopene: Lycopene is a powerful antioxidant found predominantly in tomatoes and tomato-based products. Research has shown that lycopene can reduce the risk of prostate cancer and slow the progression of existing cancer. Cooked tomatoes, such as in sauces and soups, are particularly high in bioavailable lycopene.

1. Omega-3 Fatty Acids: These essential fats, found in fatty fish like salmon, mackerel, and sardines, as well as flaxseeds and walnuts, possess anti-inflammatory properties. Omega-3 fatty acids can help reduce inflammation and potentially inhibit the growth of cancer cells.

2. Vitamin D: Adequate levels of vitamin D are crucial for maintaining prostate health. Vitamin D can be obtained through exposure to sunlight and consumption of fortified foods, fatty fish, and eggs. Studies suggest that vitamin D

may help prevent the development and progression of prostate cancer.

3. Vitamin E and Selenium: These antioxidants play a role in protecting cells from oxidative damage. Nuts, seeds, green leafy vegetables, and whole grains are excellent sources of vitamin E, while selenium is found in Brazil nuts, seafood, and brown rice.

4. Zinc: The prostate gland contains high levels of zinc, which is essential for its proper functioning. Zinc can help regulate cell growth and apoptosis (programmed cell death). Foods rich in zinc include oysters, beef, pumpkin seeds, and lentils.

5. Cruciferous Vegetables: Vegetables like broccoli, cauliflower, Brussels sprouts, and kale contain compounds that support detoxification and may reduce cancer risk. These vegetables are high in fiber, vitamins, and minerals, making them excellent additions to a prostate-healthy diet.

6. Soy Isoflavones: Found in soy products like tofu, tempeh, and soy milk, isoflavones have been shown to inhibit the growth of prostate cancer cells. Including moderate amounts of soy in the diet can be beneficial.

Foods to Include and Avoid

Knowing which foods to include and which to avoid is crucial for optimizing prostate health. Making informed choices can have a significant impact on both prevention and recovery.

Foods to Include

1. Fruits and Vegetables: Aim to consume a variety of colorful fruits and vegetables daily. Berries, citrus fruits, leafy greens, and cruciferous vegetables are particularly beneficial due to their high antioxidant content.

2. Whole Grains: Opt for whole grains like brown rice, quinoa, barley, and oats over refined grains. Whole grains provide fiber, vitamins, and minerals essential for overall health.

3. Lean Proteins: Include sources of lean protein such as poultry, fish, legumes, and plant-based proteins like tofu and tempeh. These proteins are less likely to promote inflammation compared to red and processed meats.

4. Healthy Fats: Incorporate healthy fats from sources like olive oil, avocados, nuts, and seeds. These fats support heart health and provide anti-inflammatory benefits.

5. Herbs and Spices: Use herbs and spices like turmeric, ginger, garlic, and oregano to flavor meals. These ingredients have anti-inflammatory and antioxidant properties.

Foods to Avoid

1. Red and Processed Meats: High consumption of red meat (beef, pork, lamb) and processed meats (sausages, bacon, deli meats) is linked to an increased risk of prostate cancer. Limit these foods and choose leaner protein sources instead.

2. High-Fat Dairy Products: Full-fat dairy products such as whole milk, cheese, and butter may increase the risk of prostate cancer. Opt for low-fat or plant-based alternatives.

3. Sugary Foods and Beverages: Foods and drinks high in refined sugars can contribute to obesity and inflammation, both of which are risk factors for prostate cancer. Reduce intake of sugary snacks, desserts, and sugary drinks.

4. Trans Fats: Found in many processed and fried foods, trans fats can promote inflammation and should be avoided. Check food labels for partially hydrogenated oils and avoid products containing them.

The Importance of Antioxidants and Phytochemicals

Antioxidants and phytochemicals play a crucial role in protecting cells from damage caused by free radicals and supporting overall prostate health. These compounds are abundant in plant-based foods and have been shown to have cancer-fighting properties.

Antioxidants are molecules that neutralize free radicals, which are unstable atoms that can damage cells and lead to cancer. Key antioxidants include:

1. Lycopene: Found in tomatoes, watermelon, and pink grapefruit.

2. Vitamin C: Abundant in citrus fruits, strawberries, and bell peppers.

3. Vitamin E: Present in nuts, seeds, and green leafy vegetables.

4. Beta-Carotene: Found in carrots, sweet potatoes, and spinach.

Phytochemicals are naturally occurring compounds in plants that have protective health benefits. Important phytochemicals for prostate health include:

1. Flavonoids: Found in berries, apples, onions, and tea.

2. Polyphenols: Present in green tea, grapes, and dark chocolate.

3. Sulforaphane: Found in cruciferous vegetables like broccoli and Brussels sprouts.

4. Isoflavones: Found in soy products.

5. Incorporating a variety of antioxidant- and phytochemical-rich foods into the diet can help reduce the risk of prostate cancer and support overall health.

Creating Balanced Meals

Creating balanced meals is essential for ensuring that all nutritional needs are met and for supporting prostate health. Here are some guidelines for constructing well-balanced meals:

1. Incorporate a Variety of Food Groups: Aim to include a mix of vegetables, fruits, whole grains, lean proteins, and healthy fats in each meal. This ensures a diverse intake of nutrients and helps maintain interest in meals.

2. Focus on Portion Sizes: Keep portion sizes in check to avoid overeating. Use the plate method as a guide: fill half your plate with vegetables and fruits, a quarter with lean protein, and a quarter with whole grains.

3. Balance Macronutrients: Ensure a balance of carbohydrates, proteins, and fats. Carbohydrates should come primarily from whole grains and vegetables, proteins from lean sources, and fats from healthy sources like olive oil, nuts, and avocados.

4. Stay Hydrated: Drink plenty of water throughout the day. Herbal teas and water-rich foods like fruits and vegetables can also contribute to hydration.

5. Mindful Eating: Practice mindful eating by paying attention to hunger and fullness cues. Eat slowly, savor your food, and avoid distractions like watching TV during meals.

Sample Balanced Meal:

Breakfast: Greek yogurt with fresh berries, a sprinkle of flaxseeds, and a drizzle of honey; a whole-grain toast with avocado spread.

1. Lunch: A salad with mixed greens, cherry tomatoes, cucumbers, grilled chicken breast, and a dressing made with olive oil and lemon juice; a side of quinoa.

2. Dinner: Baked salmon with a side of roasted Brussels sprouts and sweet potatoes; a mixed vegetable stir-fry with tofu and brown rice.

3. Snacks: Fresh fruit, a handful of almonds, or sliced vegetables with hummus.

By following these nutritional guidelines and creating balanced meals, individuals can support their prostate health and overall well-being. A thoughtful approach to diet, emphasizing nutrient-dense foods and mindful eating practices, can make a significant difference in preventing prostate cancer and aiding recovery.

Breakfast Recipes for Prostate Health

Nutritious Smoothies and Shakes

Smoothies and shakes are an excellent way to kickstart your day with a nutritious boost. Packed with vitamins, minerals, and antioxidants, these drinks are easy to prepare and can be tailored to support prostate health.

Berry-Lycopene Smoothie:

1. 1 cup frozen mixed berries (blueberries, strawberries, raspberries)

2. 1 ripe banana

3. 1 cup unsweetened almond milk

4. 1 tablespoon chia seeds

5. 1 handful of fresh spinach

6. 1 teaspoon honey (optional)

Instructions

1. Blend all ingredients until smooth. Berries are rich in antioxidants, while spinach provides a dose of vitamins and minerals. Chia seeds add omega-3 fatty acids and fiber, supporting overall health.

Green Power Shake:

1. 1 cup unsweetened green tea (cooled)

2. 1 small cucumber, chopped

3. 1/2 avocado

4. 1 handful of kale

5. 1 green apple, cored and sliced

6. Juice of 1/2 lemon

7. 1 tablespoon flaxseeds

Instructions

1. Blend until smooth. This shake is packed with antioxidants from green tea and kale, while avocado provides healthy fats and fiber. The apple and lemon juice add a refreshing flavor.

Whole-Grain and High-Fiber Breakfast Options

Whole grains and high-fiber foods are essential for digestive health and can help reduce the risk of prostate cancer by promoting regular bowel movements and reducing inflammation.

Overnight Oats:
1. 1/2 cup rolled oats
2. 1/2 cup unsweetened almond milk
3. 1/2 cup Greek yogurt
4. 1 tablespoon chia seeds
5. 1/2 cup fresh or frozen berries
6. 1 teaspoon honey (optional)

Instructions

1. Combine all ingredients in a jar or bowl, stir well, and refrigerate overnight. In the morning, enjoy a delicious and fiber-rich breakfast. Oats provide soluble fiber, while Greek yogurt adds protein and probiotics for gut health.

Quinoa Breakfast Bowl:

1. 1 cup cooked quinoa

2. 1/2 cup unsweetened almond milk

3. 1 tablespoon almond butter

4. 1/2 banana, sliced

5. 1 tablespoon chopped nuts (almonds, walnuts)

6. 1 teaspoon cinnamon

Instructions

1. Mix cooked quinoa with almond milk and almond butter. Top with banana slices, chopped nuts, and a sprinkle of cinnamon. Quinoa is a whole grain rich in protein and fiber, making it a satisfying and nutritious breakfast option.

Protein-Packed Morning Meals

Starting the day with a protein-packed meal can help maintain muscle mass, support metabolism, and keep you feeling full longer. These recipes offer a healthy dose of protein to support prostate health.

Vegetable Omelette:

1. 2 eggs or 3 egg whites

2. 1/4 cup diced tomatoes

3. 1/4 cup chopped spinach

4. 1/4 cup diced bell peppers

5. 1 tablespoon grated Parmesan cheese

6. 1 teaspoon olive oil

Instructions

1. Whisk eggs in a bowl. Heat olive oil in a non-stick skillet over medium heat. Add tomatoes, spinach, and bell peppers, and sauté for 2-3 minutes. Pour in the eggs and cook until set. Sprinkle with Parmesan cheese before serving. Eggs provide high-quality protein, while vegetables add vitamins and antioxidants.

Greek Yogurt Parfait:

1. 1 cup Greek yogurt

2. 1/2 cup granola (preferably low-sugar)

3. 1/2 cup mixed berries

4. 1 tablespoon honey

5. 1 tablespoon chia seeds

Instructions

1. Layer Greek yogurt, granola, and mixed berries in a glass or bowl. Drizzle with honey and sprinkle with chia seeds. This parfait is rich in protein, antioxidants, and fiber, making it a perfect morning meal.

Quick and Easy Breakfast Ideas

For busy mornings, having quick and easy breakfast options ensures you don't skip the most important meal of the day. These recipes are nutritious and can be prepared in minutes.

Avocado Toast:

1. 1 slice whole-grain bread

2. 1/2 ripe avocado

3. 1/2 teaspoon lemon juice

4. Salt and pepper to taste

5. 1 poached egg (optional)

Instructions

1. Toast the bread. Mash the avocado with lemon juice, salt, and pepper. Spread the mixture on the toast. Top with a poached egg if desired for an extra protein boost. Avocado toast provides healthy fats, fiber, and essential nutrients.

Nut Butter Banana Wrap:

1. 1 whole-grain tortilla

2. 2 tablespoons almond or peanut butter

3. 1 banana

4. 1 teaspoon honey (optional)

5. 1/2 teaspoon cinnamon

Instructions

1. Spread nut butter on the tortilla. Place the banana in the center, drizzle with honey, and sprinkle with cinnamon. Roll up the tortilla and cut in half. This wrap is a

convenient and nutritious option, combining healthy fats, protein, and fiber.

Lunch Recipes for Prostate Health

Light and Satisfying Salads

Salads are a versatile and nutritious option for lunch, providing essential vitamins, minerals, and antioxidants. Incorporating a variety of colorful vegetables, lean proteins, and healthy fats can help support prostate health.

Spinach and Berry Salad:

1. 2 cups fresh spinach leaves

2. 1/2 cup mixed berries (blueberries, strawberries, raspberries)

3. 1/4 cup sliced almonds

4. 1/4 cup crumbled feta cheese

5. 1/2 avocado, sliced

6. 1 tablespoon balsamic vinegar

7. 1 tablespoon olive oil

8. Salt and pepper to taste

Instructions

1. Combine spinach, berries, almonds, feta cheese, and avocado in a large bowl. In a small bowl, whisk together balsamic vinegar, olive oil, salt, and pepper. Drizzle the dressing over the salad and toss gently to combine. This salad is rich in antioxidants, healthy fats, and fiber, making it a light yet satisfying lunch option.

Quinoa and Chickpea Salad:

1. 1 cup cooked quinoa

2. 1 can (15 oz) chickpeas, drained and rinsed

3. 1 cucumber, diced

4. 1 red bell pepper, diced

5. 1/4 cup chopped fresh parsley

6. Juice of 1 lemon

7. 2 tablespoons olive oil

8. Salt and pepper to taste

Instructions

1. In a large bowl, mix cooked quinoa, chickpeas, cucumber, bell pepper, and parsley. In a small bowl, whisk together lemon juice, olive oil, salt, and pepper. Pour the dressing over the salad and toss well. Quinoa and chickpeas provide plant-based protein and fiber, supporting prostate health and keeping you full throughout the afternoon.

Hearty Soups and Stews

Soups and stews are comforting and can be packed with nutrient-dense ingredients. They are an excellent way to include a variety of vegetables and lean proteins in your diet.

Lentil and Vegetable Soup:
1. 1 cup dried lentils, rinsed
2. 1 onion, chopped
3. 2 carrots, chopped
4. 2 celery stalks, chopped
5. 2 garlic cloves, minced
6. 1 can (14.5 oz) diced tomatoes
7. 4 cups vegetable broth

8. 1 teaspoon dried thyme

9. 1 teaspoon cumin

10. Salt and pepper to taste

11. 2 cups chopped kale

Instructions

1. In a large pot, sauté onion, carrots, and celery until soft. Add garlic and cook for another minute. Stir in lentils, diced tomatoes, vegetable broth, thyme, cumin, salt, and pepper. Bring to a boil, then reduce heat and simmer for 30-35 minutes, or until lentils are tender. Add chopped kale and cook for an additional 5 minutes. This soup is high in fiber, protein, and essential nutrients, promoting prostate health.

Chicken and Barley Stew:

1. 2 boneless, skinless chicken breasts, diced

2. 1 onion, chopped

3. 3 carrots, sliced

4. 2 celery stalks, sliced

5. 1 cup pearl barley

6. 4 cups chicken broth

7. 1 teaspoon dried rosemary

8. 1 teaspoon dried thyme

9. Salt and pepper to taste

10. 2 cups chopped spinach

Instructions

1. In a large pot, sauté onion, carrots, and celery until soft. Add diced chicken and cook until no longer pink. Stir in barley, chicken broth, rosemary, thyme, salt, and pepper. Bring to a boil, then reduce heat and simmer for 45-50 minutes, or until barley is tender. Add chopped spinach and cook for an additional 5 minutes. This hearty stew provides lean protein, whole grains, and a variety of vegetables.

Whole-Grain Bowls and Wraps

Whole-grain bowls and wraps are convenient and can be customized with your favorite ingredients. They offer a balance of complex carbohydrates, lean proteins, and healthy fats.

Mediterranean Grain Bowl:

1. 1 cup cooked farro or brown rice

2. 1/2 cup cherry tomatoes, halved

3. 1/2 cup cucumber, diced

4. 1/4 cup Kalamata olives, sliced

5. 1/4 cup crumbled feta cheese

6. 1/4 cup hummus

7. 1 tablespoon olive oil

8. Juice of 1/2 lemon

9. Salt and pepper to taste

Instructions

1. Layer cooked farro or brown rice in a bowl. Top with cherry tomatoes, cucumber, olives, feta cheese, and a dollop of hummus. Drizzle with olive oil and lemon juice, then season with salt and pepper. This bowl is rich in fiber, antioxidants, and healthy fats, supporting prostate health and providing lasting energy.

Turkey and Avocado Wrap:

1. 1 whole-grain tortilla

2. 3-4 slices of lean turkey breast

3. 1/2 avocado, sliced

4. 1/4 cup shredded lettuce

5. 1/4 cup sliced tomatoes

6. 1 tablespoon Dijon mustard

Instructions

1. Spread Dijon mustard on the tortilla. Layer turkey, avocado, lettuce, and tomatoes. Roll up the tortilla and slice in half. This wrap is quick, easy, and packed with lean protein, healthy fats, and vitamins.

Nutrient-Dense Vegetarian and Vegan Options

Vegetarian and vegan meals can be nutrient-dense and delicious, providing essential vitamins, minerals, and antioxidants for prostate health.

Stuffed Bell Peppers:

1. 4 bell peppers, tops cut off and seeds removed

2. 1 cup cooked quinoa

3. 1 can (15 oz) black beans, drained and rinsed

4. 1 cup corn kernels

5. 1 cup diced tomatoes

6. 1/4 cup chopped cilantro

7. 1 teaspoon cumin

8. 1 teaspoon chili powder

9. Salt and pepper to taste

Instructions

1. Preheat oven to 375°F (190°C). In a large bowl, combine cooked quinoa, black beans, corn, diced tomatoes, cilantro, cumin, chili powder, salt, and pepper. Stuff the mixture into the bell peppers. Place the stuffed peppers in a baking dish and bake for 30-35 minutes, or until the peppers are tender. This vegetarian dish is high in protein, fiber, and antioxidants.

Chickpea and Spinach Curry:

1. 1 can (15 oz) chickpeas, drained and rinsed

2. 1 onion, chopped

3. 2 garlic cloves, minced

4. 1 tablespoon grated ginger

5. 1 can (14.5 oz) diced tomatoes

6. 1 can (13.5 oz) coconut milk

7. 4 cups fresh spinach

8. 1 tablespoon curry powder

9. Salt and pepper to taste

10. Cooked brown rice for serving

Instructions

1. In a large pot, sauté onion until soft. Add garlic and ginger and cook for another minute. Stir in chickpeas, diced tomatoes, coconut milk, curry powder, salt, and pepper. Bring to a simmer and cook for 15-20 minutes. Add fresh spinach and cook until wilted. Serve over cooked brown rice. This vegan curry is rich in protein, fiber, and healthy fats, making it a nutrient-dense lunch option.

Dinner Recipes for Prostate Health

Flavorful and Balanced Dinner Plates

Creating flavorful and balanced dinner plates is essential for ensuring that you get a variety of nutrients to support overall health, including prostate health. A well-balanced dinner includes a mix of lean proteins, whole grains, and plenty of vegetables.

Grilled Chicken with Quinoa and Roasted Vegetables:

1. 2 boneless, skinless chicken breasts

2. 1 cup cooked quinoa

3. 1 red bell pepper, sliced

4. 1 zucchini, sliced

5. 1 red onion, sliced

6. 2 tablespoons olive oil

7. 1 teaspoon dried oregano

8. 1 teaspoon garlic powder

9. Salt and pepper to taste

Instructions

1. Preheat the grill to medium-high heat. Season the chicken breasts with oregano, garlic powder, salt, and pepper. Grill the chicken for 6-7 minutes on each side, or until cooked through. Meanwhile, toss the bell pepper, zucchini, and red onion with olive oil, salt, and pepper. Roast the vegetables in a preheated oven at 400°F (200°C)

for 20-25 minutes, or until tender. Serve the grilled chicken over a bed of quinoa with the roasted vegetables on the side. This meal is balanced and rich in protein, fiber, and antioxidants.

Lean Protein and Vegetable Combinations

Combining lean proteins with a variety of vegetables creates meals that are not only delicious but also packed with essential nutrients. These combinations help reduce inflammation and support prostate health.

Baked Salmon with Asparagus and Sweet Potatoes:

1. 2 salmon fillets

2. 1 bunch of asparagus, trimmed

3. 2 medium sweet potatoes, cubed

4. 2 tablespoons olive oil

5. 1 teaspoon dried dill

6. 1 teaspoon garlic powder

7. Juice of 1 lemon

8. Salt and pepper to taste

Instructions

1. Preheat the oven to 400°F (200°C). Place the sweet potato cubes on a baking sheet, drizzle with olive oil, and season with salt and pepper. Roast for 15 minutes. Add the asparagus to the baking sheet, drizzle with olive oil, and season with salt and pepper. Place the salmon fillets on top of the vegetables, drizzle with olive oil, lemon juice, dill, garlic powder, salt, and pepper. Roast for an additional 15-20 minutes, or until the salmon is cooked through and the vegetables are tender. This meal provides a good source of omega-3 fatty acids, vitamins, and minerals.

Heart-Healthy Seafood Recipes

Seafood is an excellent source of lean protein and healthy fats, particularly omega-3 fatty acids, which are beneficial for heart and prostate health. Including seafood in your dinner repertoire can be both delicious and health-promoting.

Shrimp Stir-Fry with Broccoli and Bell Peppers:
1. 1 pound large shrimp, peeled and deveined

2. 1 head of broccoli, cut into florets

3. 1 red bell pepper, sliced

4. 1 yellow bell pepper, sliced

5. 2 tablespoons soy sauce (low-sodium)

6. 1 tablespoon sesame oil

7. 1 tablespoon grated ginger

8. 2 garlic cloves, minced

9. 1 tablespoon sesame seeds (optional)

10. Cooked brown rice for serving

Instructions

1. In a large skillet or wok, heat sesame oil over medium-high heat. Add ginger and garlic, and sauté for 1 minute. Add broccoli and bell peppers, and stir-fry for 5-7 minutes until tender-crisp. Add shrimp and soy sauce, and cook until the shrimp are pink and opaque, about 3-4 minutes. Sprinkle with sesame seeds if desired. Serve over cooked brown rice. This stir-fry is rich in protein, antioxidants, and healthy fats.

Plant-Based Dinner Ideas

Plant-based dinners are not only beneficial for prostate health but also for overall well-being. These recipes focus on nutrient-dense ingredients that provide essential vitamins, minerals, and antioxidants.

Lentil and Vegetable Stir-Fry:

1. 1 cup cooked lentils

2. 1 cup sliced mushrooms

3. 1 red bell pepper, sliced

4. 1 cup snap peas

5. 1 carrot, julienned

6. 2 tablespoons olive oil

7. 2 tablespoons soy sauce (low-sodium)

8. 1 tablespoon rice vinegar

9. 1 teaspoon sesame oil

10. 1 tablespoon sesame seeds (optional)

11. Cooked brown rice or quinoa for serving

Instructions

1. In a large skillet or wok, heat olive oil over medium-high heat. Add mushrooms, bell pepper, snap peas, and carrot,

and stir-fry for 5-7 minutes until tender. Add cooked lentils, soy sauce, rice vinegar, and sesame oil, and stir to combine. Cook for an additional 2-3 minutes. Sprinkle with sesame seeds if desired. Serve over cooked brown rice or quinoa. This plant-based stir-fry is high in protein, fiber, and antioxidants, making it a perfect dinner option for supporting prostate health.

Stuffed Portobello Mushrooms:

1. 4 large Portobello mushrooms, stems removed

2. 1 cup cooked quinoa

3. 1/2 cup diced tomatoes

4. 1/4 cup chopped fresh basil

5. 1/4 cup grated Parmesan cheese

6. 2 tablespoons olive oil

7. Salt and pepper to taste

Instructions

1. Preheat the oven to 375°F (190°C). Place the mushrooms on a baking sheet and brush with olive oil. In a bowl, mix cooked quinoa, diced tomatoes, chopped basil, Parmesan cheese, salt, and pepper. Stuff the mushroom caps with the

quinoa mixture. Bake for 20-25 minutes, or until the mushrooms are tender and the stuffing is golden brown. These stuffed mushrooms are a flavorful and nutritious plant-based dinner option, providing protein, fiber, and antioxidants.

Snacks and Small Bites

Healthy and Tasty Snack Options

Snacking can be a healthy and enjoyable part of your diet, especially when you choose options that provide essential nutrients and support overall health. Selecting snacks that are low in added sugars and unhealthy fats but high in fiber, protein, and healthy fats can help keep you satisfied between meals.

Apple Slices with Almond Butter:

1. 1 medium apple, sliced

2. 2 tablespoons almond butter

Apples are rich in fiber and vitamins, while almond butter provides healthy fats and protein. This combination not only satisfies your hunger but also provides a balanced mix of nutrients.

Greek Yogurt with Berries:

1. 1 cup plain Greek yogurt

2. 1/2 cup mixed berries (blueberries, strawberries, raspberries)

3. 1 teaspoon honey (optional)

Greek yogurt is an excellent source of protein and probiotics, which support digestive health. Berries are packed with antioxidants, vitamins, and fiber. This snack is both delicious and nutritious, perfect for curbing hunger between meals.

Antioxidant-Rich Snack Ideas

Antioxidants play a crucial role in protecting the body against damage from free radicals, which can contribute to chronic diseases, including cancer. Incorporating antioxidant-rich snacks into your diet can help support overall health and well-being.

Dark Chocolate and Nuts:

1. 1 ounce dark chocolate (70% cocoa or higher)

2. 1/4 cup mixed nuts (almonds, walnuts, pecans)

Dark chocolate is high in antioxidants, particularly flavonoids, which have been shown to support heart and brain health. Nuts are rich in healthy fats, protein, and additional antioxidants. This snack is satisfying and offers a powerful antioxidant boost.

Edamame with Sea Salt:

1. 1 cup edamame (fresh or frozen)

2. 1/2 teaspoon sea salt

Edamame is a great source of plant-based protein and antioxidants like isoflavones, which have been associated with various health benefits, including cancer prevention. This simple snack is easy to prepare and enjoy.

Quick and Easy Snack Prep

When you're short on time, having quick and easy snacks on hand can help you avoid less healthy options. These snacks are simple to prepare and pack, making them ideal for busy days.

Hummus and Veggie Sticks:
1. 1/2 cup hummus
2. 1 cup assorted veggie sticks (carrots, celery, bell peppers, cucumber)

Hummus is made from chickpeas, which are rich in protein and fiber. Pairing hummus with colorful veggie sticks makes for a nutritious and easy-to-prepare snack. Simply portion out the hummus and chop the veggies ahead of time for a grab-and-go option.

Hard-Boiled Eggs:
1. 2 hard-boiled eggs

Hard-boiled eggs are a convenient and protein-packed snack. They are easy to prepare in advance and can be seasoned with a pinch of salt and pepper for added flavor. Eggs provide essential amino acids and healthy fats, making them an excellent snack choice.

Energy-Boosting Small Bites

For times when you need a quick energy boost, choosing snacks that provide a balance of carbohydrates, protein, and healthy fats can help maintain your energy levels without causing a spike in blood sugar.

Energy Balls:
1. 1 cup rolled oats
2. 1/2 cup almond butter
3. 1/3 cup honey or maple syrup
4. 1/2 cup dark chocolate chips or raisins
5. 1/4 cup chia seeds or flaxseeds

Mix all ingredients in a bowl until well combined. Roll the mixture into small balls and refrigerate for at least 30 minutes. These energy balls are packed with protein, fiber, and healthy fats, making them an ideal snack to keep you energized throughout the day.

Trail Mix:

1. 1/2 cup almonds
2. 1/2 cup walnuts
3. 1/2 cup dried cranberries
4. 1/2 cup dark chocolate chips
5. 1/4 cup pumpkin seeds

Combine all ingredients in a container or bag. This homemade trail mix is a great source of healthy fats, protein, and antioxidants. It's easy to pack and enjoy as a quick, energy-boosting snack.

Desserts and Sweet Treats

Low-Sugar Dessert Options

Enjoying dessert doesn't have to mean consuming excessive sugar. Low-sugar desserts can be just as satisfying while supporting a healthy diet.

Greek Yogurt Parfait:

1. 1 cup plain Greek yogurt

2. 1/2 cup mixed berries (blueberries, strawberries, raspberries)

3. 1 tablespoon chia seeds

4. 1 teaspoon honey (optional)

Layer Greek yogurt with fresh berries and a sprinkle of chia seeds. Drizzle with honey if desired. This parfait is naturally sweet from the berries and provides protein, probiotics, and fiber, making it a nutritious and delicious low-sugar dessert.

Chocolate Avocado Mousse:

1. 2 ripe avocados

2. 1/4 cup unsweetened cocoa powder

3. 1/4 cup almond milk

4. 2-3 tablespoons honey or maple syrup

5. 1 teaspoon vanilla extract

Blend all ingredients until smooth. Refrigerate for at least 30 minutes before serving. The avocado makes this mousse creamy and rich while providing healthy fats. The cocoa powder and honey create a decadent but low-sugar treat.

Fruit-Based Desserts

Fruit-based desserts are naturally sweet and provide essential vitamins, minerals, and fiber. They can be a refreshing end to any meal.

Baked Apples with Cinnamon:
1. 4 medium apples, cored
2. 1/4 cup chopped nuts (walnuts, pecans)
3. 2 tablespoons raisins or dried cranberries
4. 1 teaspoon ground cinnamon
5. 1 tablespoon honey (optional)

Preheat the oven to 375°F (190°C). Stuff the apples with chopped nuts and dried fruit. Sprinkle with cinnamon and drizzle with honey if using. Place the apples in a baking dish and bake for 25-30 minutes, or until tender. These baked apples are warm, comforting, and naturally sweet.

Mango Coconut Chia Pudding:

1. 1 cup coconut milk

2. 1/2 cup mango puree

3. 1/4 cup chia seeds

4. 1 teaspoon vanilla extract

In a bowl, combine coconut milk, mango puree, chia seeds, and vanilla extract. Stir well and refrigerate for at least 4 hours or overnight. The chia seeds will swell and create a pudding-like consistency. This dessert is tropical, creamy, and packed with nutrients.

Baking with Healthier Ingredients

Using healthier ingredients in baking can make your desserts more nutritious without compromising taste.

Almond Flour Brownies:

1. 1 cup almond flour

2. 1/2 cup unsweetened cocoa powder

3. 1/2 cup honey or maple syrup

4. 1/4 cup coconut oil, melted

5. 2 eggs

6. 1 teaspoon vanilla extract

7. 1/2 teaspoon baking powder

8. 1/4 teaspoon salt

Preheat the oven to 350°F (175°C). In a bowl, combine almond flour, cocoa powder, baking powder, and salt. In another bowl, whisk together honey, coconut oil, eggs, and vanilla extract. Mix the wet and dry ingredients until well combined. Pour the batter into a greased baking dish and bake for 20-25 minutes. These brownies are rich and chocolatey, made with almond flour for a boost of protein and healthy fats.

Indulgent Yet Nutritious Treats

Indulgent desserts can still be nutritious by focusing on quality ingredients and balanced portions.

Dark Chocolate Covered Strawberries:

1. 1 cup dark chocolate chips (70% cocoa or higher)

2. 1 tablespoon coconut oil

3. 1 pint fresh strawberries

Melt dark chocolate chips and coconut oil together in a microwave or double boiler. Dip each strawberry into the melted chocolate, letting any excess drip off. Place the strawberries on a parchment-lined baking sheet and refrigerate until the chocolate is set. These strawberries are an elegant and indulgent treat, rich in antioxidants and vitamins.

Peanut Butter Banana Ice Cream:
1. 4 ripe bananas, sliced and frozen
2. 2 tablespoons natural peanut butter
3. 1 teaspoon vanilla extract

Blend the frozen banana slices until they reach a smooth, ice cream-like consistency. Add peanut butter and vanilla extract, blending until well combined. Serve immediately or freeze for a firmer texture. This ice cream is creamy, naturally sweet, and packed with potassium and healthy fats.

Beverages for Prostate Health

Hydrating and Healing Drinks

Staying hydrated is essential for overall health, including prostate health. Opting for hydrating beverages that also offer healing benefits can support your well-being.

Water with Lemon:

1. Plain water with a squeeze of fresh lemon juice

Water is the best choice for hydration, supporting kidney function and overall bodily functions. Adding lemon not only enhances the flavor but also provides vitamin C and antioxidants, which can help combat inflammation and support immune health.

Herbal Teas:

1. Peppermint tea, chamomile tea, or ginger tea

Herbal teas are hydrating and can offer soothing effects. Peppermint tea may help alleviate digestive issues, while chamomile tea has anti-inflammatory properties. Ginger tea can aid digestion and reduce inflammation. These teas are caffeine-free and can be enjoyed throughout the day for their calming and healing benefits.

Antioxidant-Rich Teas and Infusions

Antioxidants play a crucial role in reducing oxidative stress and inflammation, which are important considerations for prostate health. Choosing antioxidant-rich teas and infusions can provide additional health benefits.

Green Tea:

Green tea is rich in catechins, a type of antioxidant that may help reduce inflammation and protect cells from damage. It has been studied for its potential benefits in reducing the risk of prostate cancer and supporting overall prostate health.

Pomegranate Juice:

Pomegranate juice is high in antioxidants, particularly punicalagins and anthocyanins, which have anti-inflammatory properties. Studies suggest that pomegranate juice may help slow the progression of prostate cancer and improve prostate health.

Smoothies and Juices for Nutrient Boost

Smoothies and juices can be excellent ways to pack a variety of nutrients into one refreshing drink, supporting overall health and prostate function.

Berry Spinach Smoothie:
1. 1 cup mixed berries (blueberries, strawberries, raspberries)
2. 1 cup fresh spinach leaves
3. 1/2 cup plain Greek yogurt
4. 1 tablespoon chia seeds
5. 1 cup almond milk

Blend all ingredients until smooth. Berries are rich in antioxidants and fiber, while spinach provides vitamins and minerals. Greek yogurt adds protein and probiotics, and chia seeds contribute healthy fats and fiber. This smoothie is nutrient-dense and supports prostate health.

Carrot Orange Ginger Juice:

1. 4 large carrots, peeled and chopped

2. 2 oranges, peeled and segmented

3. 1-inch piece of fresh ginger, peeled

Juice the carrots, oranges, and ginger together. Carrots are high in beta-carotene, which is converted into vitamin A, essential for immune function and vision. Oranges provide vitamin C and antioxidants, while ginger has anti-inflammatory properties. This juice is refreshing and packed with immune-boosting nutrients.

Alcohol: Moderation and Health Considerations

Moderation is key when it comes to consuming alcohol, as excessive intake can negatively impact prostate health and overall well-being.

Red Wine:

Red wine contains antioxidants, such as resveratrol, which may have protective effects on cardiovascular health. Some studies suggest that moderate consumption of red wine may also benefit prostate health. However, it's important to limit alcohol intake to no more than one drink per day for women and two drinks per day for men, as excessive alcohol consumption can increase the risk of prostate cancer and other health problems.
Water with Cranberry Juice:

Mix cranberry juice with water for a refreshing drink that also provides antioxidants and potential urinary tract health benefits. Cranberry juice contains compounds that may help prevent urinary tract infections, which can be beneficial for prostate health.

Meal Plans and Tips for Success

Weekly Meal Plans for Prostate Health

Creating a weekly meal plan tailored to prostate health can help you maintain a balanced diet rich in nutrients that support overall well-being.

Day 1:

Breakfast: Nutritious Smoothie with berries, spinach, Greek yogurt, and chia seeds.
Lunch: Quinoa Salad with grilled chicken, mixed greens, cherry tomatoes, and avocado.
Dinner: Baked Salmon with asparagus and sweet potatoes.
Snack: Greek yogurt with mixed berries.

Day 2:

Breakfast: Oatmeal topped with sliced bananas, nuts, and a drizzle of honey.

Lunch: Lentil and Vegetable Stir-Fry.

Dinner: Stuffed Portobello Mushrooms with quinoa and vegetable filling.

Snack: Apple slices with almond butter.

Shopping Lists and Pantry Staples

Having a well-stocked pantry and shopping list can streamline meal preparation and ensure you have essential ingredients on hand.

Pantry Staples:

Whole grains: Quinoa, brown rice, oats.

Protein sources: Canned beans (e.g., black beans, chickpeas), lentils, canned tuna or salmon.

Healthy fats: Olive oil, coconut oil, nuts (almonds, walnuts).

Herbs and spices: Garlic powder, turmeric, basil, oregano.

Snacks: Mixed nuts, seeds (chia seeds, flaxseeds), whole-grain crackers.

Shopping List:

Fresh produce: Leafy greens (spinach, kale), colorful vegetables (bell peppers, broccoli), fruits (berries, apples, bananas).

Lean proteins: Chicken breasts, salmon fillets, tofu.

Dairy and alternatives: Greek yogurt, almond milk.

Whole grains: Quinoa, brown rice.

Miscellaneous: Eggs, honey or maple syrup (for sweeteners), dark chocolate (70% cocoa or higher).

Meal Prep and Batch Cooking Tips

Efficient meal prep and batch cooking can save time and ensure you have healthy meals readily available throughout the week.

1. Plan Ahead: Create a weekly meal plan and shopping list based on recipes you want to try.

2. Prep Ingredients: Wash and chop vegetables, cook grains, and portion out snacks ahead of time.

3. Batch Cooking: Prepare large batches of staples like quinoa, roasted vegetables, and grilled chicken to use in multiple meals.

4. Storage: Use airtight containers or meal prep containers to store prepared ingredients and meals in the refrigerator or freezer.

Strategies for Staying on Track

Staying consistent with your meal plan and healthy eating goals is essential for long-term success.

1. Set Realistic Goals: Start with achievable goals and gradually incorporate healthier choices into your diet.

2. Stay Organized: Use a meal planner or app to schedule meals and track progress.

3. Practice Mindful Eating: Pay attention to hunger and fullness cues, and avoid distractions while eating.

4. Stay Hydrated: Drink plenty of water throughout the day to support digestion and overall health.

5. Seek Support: Share your goals with friends or family members who can encourage and support your journey.

By following a structured meal plan, stocking up on essential ingredients, mastering meal prep techniques, and implementing strategies for consistency, you can optimize your diet for prostate health and overall well-being. Remember to enjoy variety in your meals and listen to your body's needs for sustained success.

Lifestyle and Dietary Tips for Prostate Cancer Patients

Living with prostate cancer involves adopting lifestyle and dietary strategies that can support overall health and well-being, alongside medical treatment. Here are key tips to consider:

The Importance of Regular Exercise

Regular physical activity is crucial for prostate cancer patients as it offers numerous health benefits:

1. Strength and Endurance: Exercise helps maintain muscle strength and endurance, which can support overall physical function during treatment.

2. Bone Health: Weight-bearing exercises like walking or strength training can help maintain bone density, which may be affected by certain treatments.

3. Mood and Well-being: Physical activity can reduce symptoms of depression and anxiety, common among cancer patients, by promoting the release of endorphins.

4. Immune Function: Regular exercise can strengthen the immune system, potentially aiding in recovery and reducing the risk of infections.

5. Prostate cancer patients should aim for at least 150 minutes of moderate-intensity aerobic exercise per week, such as brisk walking, swimming, or cycling, along with strength training exercises two days a week.

Stress Management Techniques

Managing stress is essential for coping with the emotional and psychological challenges of prostate cancer:

1. Mindfulness and Meditation: Practices like mindfulness meditation or deep-breathing exercises can help reduce stress and promote relaxation.

2. Yoga or Tai Chi: These mind-body practices combine gentle movements with breath awareness, aiding in stress reduction and improving flexibility.

3. Support Groups: Joining a support group for cancer patients can provide emotional support, shared experiences, and practical coping strategies.

4. Finding effective stress management techniques can improve quality of life and enhance overall well-being during and after prostate cancer treatment.

The Role of Supplements

While a balanced diet should provide most essential nutrients, some prostate cancer patients may benefit from specific supplements:

1. Vitamin D: Many cancer patients have low vitamin D levels, which may impact immune function and bone health. Consult with a healthcare provider to determine appropriate supplementation.

2. Omega-3 Fatty Acids: These healthy fats, found in fish oil supplements, may have anti-inflammatory properties beneficial for overall health.

3. Probiotics: Supporting gut health with probiotic supplements or foods like yogurt may help manage digestive issues often associated with cancer treatment.

4. Always consult with a healthcare provider before starting any new supplements to ensure they are safe and appropriate for your individual health needs.

Building a Supportive Eating Environment

Creating a supportive eating environment can positively impact nutritional intake and overall health:

1. Meal Planning: Plan and prepare meals ahead of time to ensure nutritious options are readily available, making it easier to maintain a balanced diet.

2. Family and Social Support: Engage family members and friends in meal preparation and eating together, fostering a supportive environment.

3. Hydration: Stay hydrated by drinking water throughout the day, which is essential for overall health and may help manage certain side effects of treatment.

4. Maintaining a varied and nutrient-rich diet, focusing on whole grains, lean proteins, fruits, and vegetables, can provide essential nutrients to support immune function and overall well-being. Adjusting dietary choices to manage treatment side effects, such as nausea or changes in taste, can also improve quality of life.

Prostate Cancer Recipes

Smoky Kale Saute

This Smoky Kale Saute is a quick vegan version of the southern soul food standby that uses kale instead of collards. It makes a great side for any meal, from Roast Chicken to grilled tofu. Steaming then shocking the kale in cold water will help it to keep its gorgeous green color. The smoked paprika adds such a fabulous smoky taste that the usual ham hock won't be missed.

Ingredients

* 2 small bunches kale, washed and tough stems removed

* ½ cup water

* 1 tablespoon olive oil

* 3 cloves garlic, smashed and sliced

* ½ cup canned or fresh diced tomatoes

* ¼ teaspoon smoked paprika

* Sea salt, to taste

Directions

1. Put the kale into a pan with the water. Sprinkle with a little sea salt and cover. Bring to a boil and cook until the kale is just wilted and a dark rich green, about 3 to 5 minutes. Remove the kale and run under cold water to stop the cooking. Drain. Squeeze out any excess water, coarsely chop and set aside.

2. Heat the oil in a sauté pan over a medium heat. Add the garlic and cook until it just starts to turn golden. Add the tomatoes, sprinkle with a little sea salt and cook for 5 minutes.

3. Add the smoked paprika. Cook stirring for 1 minute. Add the kale. Stir to coat the kale with the tomato and spice. Cook until the kale has heated through. If the pan looks dry, add ¼ cup of hot water to the pan and cook stirring until it has evaporated. Serve immediately.

Quick Fish Stew

Fish is a great lean protein for a healthy survivorship. This quick fish stew is a favorite at our classes. It's easy to make and delicious to eat! Fish is so very good for us and this stew is great for beginners because it is pretty much foolproof. The stew base can be frozen, too — check out the Chef Tips. You can even cook the potatoes and carrots ahead of time to add to the stew along with the fish — just make sure they are al dente, which means that they still have some bite.

Ingredients

* 1 pound firm white fish fillets (cod, hake, monkfish), skinned and cut into large pieces
* Sea salt and black pepper, to taste
* 2 teaspoons ground cumin, divided
* 2 tablespoons olive oil
* 2 cloves of garlic, thinly sliced
* 1 large onion, chopped
* 1 (14-ounce) can diced tomatoes
* 2 carrots, cut into large chunks
* 4 medium potatoes, peeled and quartered
* 3 to 4 cups low-sodium chicken or vegetable stock
* 1 cup cooked or frozen peas
* 2 tablespoons chopped cilantro

Directions

1. Rub the fish with salt and pepper to taste and half the powdered cumin. Set aside in the fridge while you prepare the stew base.

2. Heat the olive oil in a large pot over medium-high heat. Saute the garlic until it starts to color. Add the onion and saute until it softens and takes on a golden color, about 5 minutes. Add the rest of the cumin, mix with the onions and fry for a minute — do not let it burn!

3. Add a little stock to deglaze the pan. Add the tomatoes and cook them down until they start to take on an orangey color. Add the carrots and potatoes and enough stock to just cover them. Mix and cover the pan. Cook over low heat until the vegetables are just tender.

4. Add the fish, cover, and cook until it starts to turn opaque. Then add the peas and cook until the fish is done, about 2 minutes. Add the cilantro. Leave to sit, covered, for 5 minutes before you serve it. Add salt to taste. Serve the fish with the vegetables, some extra chopped cilantro, and a wedge of lime.

Broccoli Pesto

Pesto isn't always about pine nuts and basil, it can be about other members of the vegetable kingdom too, as here. Broccoli is blanched then pureed with garlic, parmesan, fresh basil, and toasted walnuts to make a super-simple nutritious sauce to toss with al dente whole-wheat pasta or to stir into rice as a condiment. Either way it's delicious.

Ingredients

* 1½ cups broccoli florets (see Ann's Tips)
* 8 ounces whole wheat fusilli pasta (2-ounces per person)
* 1 to 2 garlic cloves, minced, to taste
* 1 teaspoon salt
* ⅓ cup olive oil
* ¼ cup toasted walnuts
* ⅓ cup freshly grated Parmesan cheese
* 1 stem basil leaves

Directions

1. Bring salted water to boil in a pot. Add the broccoli and boil for 5 minutes. Drain and run under cold water.

2. In the same pot, bring another batch of salted water to boil. Cook pasta according to package instructions. Drain and reserve ¼ cup of cooking liquid.

3. In a food processor, process the salt, garlic, and olive oil until the garlic is evenly chopped. Add the drained broccoli, walnuts, Parmesan cheese, and basil. Process until well blended with some texture remaining. Taste for seasoning.

4. Cover and refrigerate pesto if not using immediately. Toss the pesto with the drained pasta, adding some cooking liquid if the pesto is too thick. Serve warm or at room temperature.

Quick Tomato Sauce

Ingredients

* 2 tablespoons olive oil

* 1 to 2 cloves garlic, smashed and thinly sliced lengthwise

* 1 small dried red chili pepper, seeds removed (optional)

* 1½ pounds ripe plum tomatoes (about 6-8), coarsely chopped (see Chef Tips)

* ¼ – ½ teaspoon brown sugar (if using canned tomatoes)

* ½ teaspoon salt, or to taste

* 1 tablespoon freshly grated Parmesan cheese (optional)

Directions

1. Heat the oil in a wok or heavy frying pan over medium-high heat. When the oil starts to shimmer, add the garlic and saute until golden. Do not let it burn or it will become bitter. If you like a spicy sauce, add the pepper.

2. Add the tomatoes and saute. There will be a lot of spitting and hissing as the wet tomatoes hit the hot oil. Turn the heat to medium-low, add the sugar if using, and cook the tomatoes down until they are reduced by about half and have taken on a more orangey hue. Adjust the seasoning by adding salt to taste. If the sauce looks like it's drying out too much, add a little water. At this point, if not using immediately, stop cooking, cool, and freeze the sauce for later use.

3. Add the Parmesan, taste for seasoning, then serve.

Roasted Broccoli

This easy, umami-rich recipe is a sure-fire way to get the broccoli haters in your life to eat this amazingly nutritious veggie. Roasting veggies brings out their natural sweetness, and broccoli is no exception. The Parmesan cheese gives it a savory and salty flavor if you end up using it.

Ingredients
* 1 pound broccoli, rinsed and dried
* 1 tablespoon olive oil
* ½ cup freshly grated Parmesan or Pecorino cheese (optional)
* Salt and pepper, to taste

Directions
1. Preheat the oven to 425 degrees.
2. Cut about 1-inch off the stalk of the broccoli. Peel the rest of the stem and cut the through the broccoli lengthwise then roughly into wedges, so you have long broccoli spears (see Chef Tips).
3. Pour the olive oil into a large bowl. Add a little salt and pepper. Add the broccoli spears and toss to coat with olive

oil, use your hands. Add the grated cheese and toss again, if using. Transfer to a parchment-lined baking sheet. Sprinkle the broccoli with any remaining cheese left in the bowl.

4. Bake for 20 minutes until broccoli is golden and crispy around edges. Serve immediately.

Lemon-Soy Baked Tofu Steaks

This delicious lemon-soy baked tofu recipe uses a Westernized version of a traditional Japanese teriyaki marinade. For really tasty tofu, the best way is to simply bake the tofu covered in marinade instead of marinating it before cooking. It is important to take the time to press the excess water out of the tofu so that it takes up as much of the marinade as possible during cooking, and doesn't dilute the marinade.

Ingredients

* 2 blocks of firm tofu, sliced into ½-inch thick slices.

Marinade:

* ⅔ cup soy sauce

* 2 teaspoon lemon, grated and zested

* 4 tablespoons lemon juice

* 2 tablespoons balsamic vinegar

* 2 teaspoons sugar

* 4 tablespoons olive oil (See Chef Tips if on a Bland Diet)

* 2 cloves garlic, crushed and sliced

* 2 tablespoon chopped fresh herbs, tarragon, rosemary or thyme (Optional)

Directions

1. Lay the tofu out on a board or tray lined with paper towels or a clean tea towel. Cover with more paper. Lay a wooden cutting board or other weight on top to press out the excess moisture so that the marinade won't be diluted. (I often use wine or water bottles as weights.) This will take about 30 minutes. It's best to do this near the sink. You will be amazed by how much water comes out.

2. Preheat the oven to 400 degrees.

3. Put all the ingredients together in a saucepan, except the herbs. Bring to a boil. Take it off the heat immediately and cool. Add the herbs once the marinade is off the heat.

4. Once the tofu is drained, pat the slices dry. Spoon a little marinade onto a lightly greased baking dish and lay the tofu

slices over it, side by side in a single layer. Pour the rest of the marinade over them. Bake uncovered for 25 minutes, turning the slices over about halfway through. The tofu should be brown and almost dry, and any remaining marinade thick and syrupy. Serve immediately!

Black Bean Chili

Ingredients

* 2 tablespoons grapeseed oil

* 2 cloves of garlic, minced

* 1 teaspoon cumin seeds

* 1 medium onion diced

* 1 poblano pepper, seeded and cut into a ½-inch dice (see Chef Tips)

* 1 bay leaf

* 1 chipotle chile in adobo, chopped into a fine paste (see Chef Tips)

* 1 cup chopped tomatoes

* 2 (14 ounce) cans drained and rinsed, or 3 cups fresh cooked black beans, broth reserved

* 1 cup stock, bean broth or water

* 3 to 4 whole sprigs cilantro, washed well

* Juice of 1 lime

* 3 tablespoons chopped cilantro, plus more for garnish

* ½ cup grated cheese, for garnish (optional)

* Sea salt and black pepper, to taste

Directions

1. Heat the oil in a large wide skillet or saute pan over medium-high heat. Add the garlic and fry until it starts to turn light gold in color, about 30 seconds to 1 minute.

2. Add the cumin seeds and fry until they darken and start to give off their aroma, about 1 minute. Take care not to let the seeds burn.

3. Add the onion, poblano pepper, and the bay leaf. Cook, stirring until the vegetables start to soften and the onion is transparent and turning golden. Add the chipotle pepper paste. Cook, stirring for about 30 seconds.

4. Add the tomatoes and cook until the tomatoes start to change to an orangey red color. Add the beans and ½ cup stock, stirring to mix. Lay the cilantro stems on top of the beans and cover. Turn the heat down to low and simmer for about 20 minutes, or until you are ready for them. Check

from time to time, and add more stock or broth if the beans look dry.

5. Remove the bay leaf and cilantro stems. Stir in the lime juice and 2 tablespoons chopped cilantro. Serve immediately with the remaining cilantro and grated cheese as a garnish.

Goat Cheese, Onion, Spinach & Lemon Pizza

Ingredients

* 1 teaspoon olive oil

* 1 clove garlic, smashed

* 2 cups packed baby spinach, washed

* 1 tablespoon panko or cornmeal

* 1 whole wheat pizza dough or refrigerated or frozen pizza crust

* ½ cup storebought tomato sauce or our Quick Tomato Sauce

* ¾ cup goat cheese

* ½ small onion, halved and thinly sliced

* ½ cup cherry tomatoes or grape tomatoes, halved

* 1 tablespoon olive oil

* Salt and pepper, to taste

* ½ a lemon, zested

Directions

1. Preheat the oven to 500 degrees F. Put 2 baking trays into the oven, or pizza stone if available.

2. In a medium sauté pan, over medium-high heat, add the 1 teaspoon of olive oil and clove of garlic. Cook until the garlic starts to brown and become fragrant. Remove the garlic and add the baby spinach along with 1 tablespoon of water. Let sit for 1 minute and then stir. Once the spinach has wilted, remove from pan and let drain. Once cool enough, squeeze out excess liquid.

3. Sprinkle panko or cornmeal onto a large sheet of parchment paper. Roll out the dough onto the parchment paper; press out dough into a 12x8-inch rectangle or to fit your pizza stone. Split into two balls if necessary.

4. Spread the tomato sauce evenly onto the dough. Dot the pizza with the goat cheese and top it with the drained spinach, onions, and grape tomatoes, cut sides up. Drizzle with olive oil and sprinkle with a little salt and pepper.

5. Using the parchment paper, slip the pizza onto the heated baking trays or pizza stone. Bake in the oven on the lowest rack for 10-15 minutes, or until the crust is golden and the cheese looks melted.

6. Using the parchment paper, slip the pizza onto a cutting board. Sprinkle with the lemon zest and cut into slices.

Watermelon Feta Salad

The tasty bite of sweet watermelon, salty cheese, and bitter arugula is really delicious. You will need a sweet, ripe melon for the best result. A good way to find that out is to tap the melon before you buy – if it sounds hollow, then it is ready to eat.

Ingredients

* 1 medium shallot or ½ small red onion, sliced very thin

* ½ cup cider vinegar

* 1 small watermelon, chilled

* 4 ounces fresh feta cheese or ricotta salata, cut or crumbled into small chunks

* 1 handful torn mint leaves

* Juice of 1 to 2 limes, or to taste

* 4 cups loosely packed arugula, rinsed

Directions

1. In a bowl combine the thinly sliced onion and vinegar. Let sit for at least 30 minutes. Drain.

2. Meanwhile, cut the melon into 8-12 slices. Cut away the rind and cut the flesh into 1-inch chunks. Put into a large bowl.

3. Mix the watermelon with half of the lime juice. Add more lime juice to taste. Let sit in the fridge to marinate and chill.

4. Just before serving, quickly toss together with the cheese and the mint. Lay arugula down on a serving platter and top with watermelon and cheese mixture, and dot the onions over the top. Serve immediately.

Spicy Sausage Pasta with Lemon & Broccoli

This Spicy Sausage Pasta with Lemon & Broccoli is traditional pasta is quick and easy, plus it's a favorite with the guys. Broccoli rabe and orrechiette pasta are classically used for this dish, but we're going to be using broccoli, chicken sausage, and a chunky whole wheat pasta. This dish is a great vehicle for healthy broccoli. It defies its bland, dull stereotype, turning it into something quite other. Just be sure to make the florets small so that they cook through quickly. Undercook the pasta by 1 minute so it can finish cooking in the sauce. In the summer, try adding 12 cup fresh, ripe, chopped tomato instead of the reserved cooking water at step 5.

Ingredients
* 1 bunch broccoli broken into small florets, washed, stems reserved
* 4 ounces whole wheat pasta (use penne, rigatoni or any other chunky pasta)
* 2 tablespoons olive oil
* 1 stalk of rosemary, leaves stripped and chopped or ½ teaspoon dried
* Pinch of dried red pepper flakes, or to taste
* 1 to 2 hot Italian style chicken sausages, squeezed out of their casings

* 1 to 2 cloves of garlic, smashed peeled and slice length ways

* 1 tablespoon grated lemon peel

* 2 tablespoons lemon juice

* 2 tablespoons freshly grated Parmesan cheese (optional)

* 1 tablespoon fresh chopped Italian parsley

* Salt and black pepper, to taste

Directions

1. Peel and thinly julienne the thick parts of the broccoli stems. Set aside.

2. Bring salt water to boil. Add pasta and cook for 1 minute less than package instructions.

3. While the water is boiling heat the oil in a heavy frying pan at medium-high heat. Add the rosemary and red pepper flakes and fry for 1 minute. Add the sausage flattening it as you fry, breaking it up into small pieces. When it starts to turn brown, add the broccoli stems and garlic. Cook until the stems start to brown. Remove from heat if the pasta is not ready yet.

4. When the pasta is ready, heat up the pan with the sausage. With a slotted spoon transfer the pasta and ¼ cup

of pasta water directly into the pan with sausage. Put the broccoli florets into the still boiling pasta water. Cook for one minute and transfer to the pan with sausage. Mix well to coat the broccoli and pasta.

5. Stir in lemon zest, juice, grated Parmesan, and then add the parsley into the sauce. Check for salt. Add a little more of the reserved water if the pan looks too dry. Grind some black pepper over it and serve with freshly grated Parmesan cheese.

Melanie's Flaxseed & Walnut Pesto

This great pesto sauce was created for a Cook for Your Life class taught by Chef Melanie Underwood. While pesto is usually made with pine nuts, this pesto offers a clever, delicious way to add omega-3-rich flaxseeds and walnuts into your diet. Toss this nutritious condiment over veggies or pasta, or stir it into brown rice or quinoa.

Ingredients
* 2 tablespoons walnuts, toasted
* 2 tablespoons flaxseeds

* 2 cups packed basil or flat leaf (Italian) parsley leaves

* 1 to 2 garlic cloves

* 3 tablespoons Parmesan cheese, freshly grated

* 2 to 4 tablespoons water

Directions

1. In a food processor, combine the walnuts and flaxseeds, process until ground, about 1-2 minutes.

2. Add basil or parsley, garlic, Parmesan, and 2 tablespoons water. Puree until smooth and thick, adding more water, a little at a time, if necessary.

Kale Chips

Kale chips are delicious. But kale can be a hard vegetable to get people to eat without some persuasion — until they try kale chips, that is. The most hardened kale naysayer will gobble them up without hesitation, even kids. Try them.

Ingredients
* 1 bunch (about 6-ounces) kale, rinsed (see Chef Tips)
* 1 tablespoon olive oil

* Salt, to taste

Directions

1. Preheat the oven to 350 degrees.

2. With a paper towel pat the kale dry. Remove stems and rip the leaves into roughly 1-inch pieces.

3. Toss the kale with olive oil and a good pinch of salt. Put onto a baking sheet and cook until the kale is crispy and dried out, about 10-12 minutes. Let cool. Store in an airtight container.

Roasted Tomato & Olive Pearl Couscous

Pearl couscous is a fabulously showy version of the pantry staple. It looks gorgeous and tastes delicious in this Roasted Tomato & Olive Pearl Couscous which is a macro version of tabbouleh that uses slow roasted instead of raw tomatoes. Slow roasting brings out the sweetness of cherry tomatoes in spades, and turns the garlic into a sweet, nutty-tasting paste that flavors the dressing. If you are on an anti-microbial regimen, cooking the tomatoes makes eating this tabbouleh salad possible. You will need to wash herbs very well to add them raw, or quickly sauté the chopped herbs in a little stock or olive oil before adding them to the salad.

Ingredients
* 2 pints (4 cups) red grape or cherry tomatoes
* 3 large garlic cloves, unpeeled
* ¼ cup extra-virgin olive oil
* ¼ cup warm water
* 1 teaspoon fresh lemon juice
* 1 teaspoon salt
* ¼ teaspoon black pepper
* 2¾ cups Chicken Broth
* 2¼ cups pearl (Israeli) couscous
* 1 tablespoon olive oil
* ½ cup Kalamata or other brine-cured black olives, pitted and chopped
* ⅓ cup chopped fresh flat-leaf parsley
* ¼ cup chopped fresh mint
* 1 teaspoon chopped fresh thyme

Directions

1. Preheat oven to 250 degrees.

2. Halve tomatoes through stem ends and arrange cut sides up, in a single layer on a large baking pan with the unpeeled garlic. Roast in the middle of oven until tomatoes are slightly shriveled around edges, about 1 hour. Cool in pan on a rack 30 minutes.

3. Squeeze roasted garlic out of its skin and puree with the olive oil, water, lemon juice, salt, pepper, and ½ cup roasted tomatoes in a blender until dressing is very smooth.

4. Bring the chicken broth to a boil in a 3-quart heavy saucepan and stir in couscous, then simmer, uncovered, 6 minutes. Cover pan and remove from heat. Let stand for 10 minutes.

5. Spread couscous in 1 layer on a baking sheet and cool 15 minutes. Transfer couscous to a bowl and stir with the pureed dressing, roasted tomatoes, olives, parsley, mint, thyme and salt and pepper to taste.

Asparagus & Goat Cheese Frittata

Frittatas are a great way to either use up vegetables for a quick supper, or to make a great centerpiece for a special breakfast or brunch. With this asparagus & goat cheese frittata, because we are using a lot of vegetables, we don't need too many eggs to make it plus, if you use eggs from free roaming hens, the frittata will be very rich and you'll find a little will go a long way!

Ingredients

* 4 large eggs

* ¼ cup water

* 1 tablespoon Parmesan cheese, freshly grated

* Salt and pepper, to taste

* 2 teaspoons extra virgin olive oil

* 1 tablespoon scallions, chopped white and light green parts only

* ½-pound asparagus, steamed and cut into ½-inch pieces, tips reserved.

* 1 medium potato, boiled and cut into a ½-inch dice

* 2-ounce fresh goat cheese, crumbled

* Olive oil or unsalted butter, as needed

Directions

1. Preheat the oven to 350 degrees.

2. In a large bowl, whisk the eggs. Gradually beat in the water. Add the Parmesan, salt and pepper to taste.

3. Heat the olive oil in a skillet over medium heat, Sauté the scallions until soft. Put the scallion mixture into the egg mixture.

4. Grease the skillet with a little butter or olive oil. Arrange the reserved asparagus tips in the bottom of the pan. Set aside.

5. Mix the remaining cut asparagus and potato pieces into the eggs and herbs. Fold in the goat cheese. Carefully pour the egg mixture over the asparagus tips in the skillet. Put the skillet in the middle of the oven and bake until the frittata is set, about 35 to 40 minutes. Let cool for 5 minutes in the pan. Turn the frittata out onto a plate to cool to room temperature. Serve with a simple green salad.

Asparagus, Lima Bean & Almond Pasta

This is an easy way to use the small green asparagus we get in the spring. It's also a great dish to make if you're feeling tired. You can literally pull it together in...

For more protein, we've added ½ cup of frozen lima beans. We have also reserved some pasta water to moisten the sauce instead of adding in more oil. Serve it with a chunk of Parmigiano on the table ready to be grated over the pasta.

Ingredients

* 3 tablespoons almonds, sliced

* 1 tablespoon sea salt, for the pasta water

* 8 ounces whole wheat rotini or penne pasta

* 1 pound green asparagus, trimmed and cut into 1-inch pieces

* 1 cup frozen baby lima beans

* 3 tablespoons olive oil

* 2 cloves garlic, smashed, peeled and thinly sliced

* 1 dried pepper pod, de-seeded (optional)

* 3 tablespoons Italian parsley, chopped

* 1 tablespoon Parmigiano Reggiano cheese, grated (optional)

* Sea salt and black pepper to taste

Directions

1. Toast the sliced almonds in a heavy- wide pan until they are just turning golden. Transfer to a bowl and set aside.

2. Bring salted water to a boil in a large pot. Add pasta to the boiling water and continue to boil for 7 minutes, or 3 minutes less than package instructions. Add the asparagus and frozen lima beans to the boiling pasta and cook for 2 minutes. Reserve 1 cup of pasta water, then drain the pasta and vegetables -- they should be a little undercooked.

3. Meanwhile, in a deep pan or wok, heat olive oil over medium-high heat. Once the oil is hot, add the garlic and chili pepper, if using. Continue cooking until the garlic is light gold, about 3 minutes. Do not let the garlic burn.

4. Add the parsley to the pan and stir-fry for 1 minute. Add ¼ cup of pasta water to the pan and bring to a simmer. Add the almonds, and turn the heat down to medium. If the pan gets dry, add more pasta water, a little at a time.

5. Add the drained pasta, asparagus, and lima beans to the pan. Stir well, and add in the remaining pasta water, stirring continuously and allowing to reduce. Add the grated cheese and a grind or two of black pepper. Mix well and cook for another minute. Taste for seasonings then serve.

Maple-Glazed Salmon

A light marinade or glaze is an easy way to liven up an everyday piece of salmon and get your omega- 3s. This dish is a subtle, Americanized version of a traditional Japanese teriyaki glaze that uses maple syrup as a sweetener, instead of sugar. With a light citrus and maple flavor, this salmon also makes for a festive dish at holiday time.

Ingredients
* ¼ cup soy sauce
* ¼ cup maple syrup
* 4 cloves garlic, smashed and sliced
* 2 tablespoons grated ginger
* 1 tablespoon orange zest
* 1-pound salmon fillet

Directions
1. In a small bowl whisk the soy sauce, maple syrup, garlic, ginger, and orange zest together.
2. Place the salmon fillet in a re-sealable plastic bag and pour in the soy mixture. Close the bag and place onto a

plate and store in the refrigerator for 30 minutes to 1 hour. (Do not marinate longer than 24 hours.)

3. Preheat your broiler. Remove the salmon from the bag and discard the garlic. Place onto a baking try and broil for 8 minutes on each side or until cooked through. Serve immediately or at room temperature.

Chicken Sausage & Kale Pizza

In this pizza recipe, we use chicken sausage instead of pepperoni and deliver a nutritional bonus with the addition of kale. You can find pre-made raw pizza dough or reheatable pizza crusts in many markets if making your own dough isn't an option.

Ingredients

* 1 tablespoon olive oil

* 3 chicken or turkey sausages, casings removed

* 1 tablespoon panko or cornmeal

* Whole-wheat pizza dough, or refrigerated or frozen pizza crust (see Chef Tips)

* ½ cup tomato sauce (see Chef Tips)

* ¾ cup mozzarella cheese, grated

* ¾ cup packed kale leaves, washed, patted dry, and torn into pieces

* ½ cup cherry or grape tomatoes, halved

* Salt and pepper to taste

Directions

1. Preheat the oven to 500 degrees. Put 2 baking trays into the oven, or pizza stone if you have one.

2. In a saute pan, heat the olive oil. Once it's hot, cook the sausages until cooked through and starting to brown. Pour onto a plate lined with a paper towel.

3. Split the dough into 4 equal balls if making personal pizzas. Sprinkle panko or cornmeal onto a large sheet of parchment paper. Roll out the dough onto the parchment paper; press out dough into a 12-by-8-inch rectangle or to fit your pizza stone. Split into two balls if necessary.

4. Spread the Quick Tomato Sauce evenly onto the dough and sprinkle with cheese. Top with kale, sausage, and grape tomatoes, cut sides up. Sprinkle with a little salt and pepper.

5. Using the parchment paper, slip the pizza onto the heated baking trays or pizza stone. Bake in the oven on the lowest rack for 10 to 15 minutes, or until the crust is golden and the cheese is bubbling.

6. Using the parchment paper, slip the pizza onto a cutting board and cut into slices. Drizzle with olive oil if desired. Serve with a simple green salad.

Eggs Baked in Tomatoes

Roasting tomatoes brings out all their natural sweetness. When beefsteak tomatoes are at their best, use them to make this easy, delicious, spectacular Eggs Baked in Tomatoes breakfast or brunch dish. No one could feel deprived for one minute eating this!

Ingredients

* 4 large tomatoes

* 2 cloves of garlic, chopped

* Olive oil

* Salt and pepper, to taste

* 4 large eggs

* 3 tablespoons Parmesan cheese

* Fresh basil, for garnish

Directions

1. Preheat the oven to 400 degrees F.

2. Slice the top quarter off of each tomato. Using a paring knife or spoon, carefully core the tomato. Transfer to a 2-inch deep baking pan lined with parchment paper. Drizzle with olive oil, salt, pepper, and some chopped garlic. Bake for 20 minutes, or until the tomatoes have broken down slightly.

3. Remove the pan from the oven and carefully crack an egg into each tomato. The egg whites will dribble out. Return to the oven and cook for another 6 to 8 minutes or until the yolks have just set (cook until completely hard if on low microbial or neutropenic diet). Top with some Parmesan cheese and return to the oven for another 1 to 2 minutes.

4. Serve warm or at room temperature with fresh basil.

Fennel & Tomato Gratin

This fennel & tomato gratin hails from the South of France and makes a wonderful side. It's quick to make and quite delicious with both fish and chicken. It's also great if cancer is in the equation, too. The tomatoes are packed with cancer-fighting lycopene, and fennel is easy on the digestive system. To cut out the dairy, just leave out the cheese from the breadcrumbs for a Mediterranean-style, vegan treat.

Ingredients

* 5 medium fennel bulbs, stalks removed (see Ann's tips)
* 1 cup homemade breadcrumbs, or to taste
* ¾ cup finely grated Parmesan cheese
* Black pepper, to taste, Freshly ground
* 2 tablespoons olive oil

For the Quick Tomato Sauce,

* 2 tablespoons olive oil
* 1 1/2 pounds ripe plum tomatoes (about 6-8), coarsely chopped (See Chef Tips)
* 1 to 2 cloves garlic, smashed and thinly sliced lengthwise
* 1 small dried red pepper, seeds removed (optional)

* 1/2 teaspoon salt or to taste

* 1 tablespoons, freshly grated Parmesan cheese (optional)

Directions

1. Preheat the oven to 350 degrees F. Prepare the quick tomato sauce as outlined here.

2. Halve the fennel bulbs and parboil in salted water for about 10 minutes or until they are just soft and slightly translucent looking. Drain. Cut into quarters. If the bulbs are very large, cut each half into 3 pieces. Set aside.

3. Toss the breadcrumbs and the cheese together in a bowl. Set aside.

4. Bring the Quick Tomato Sauce to a boil over a medium high flame in a wide sauté pan. Lower the heat to medium and simmer until the sauce has thickened, about 10 to 15 minutes. Set aside.

5. Spread a thin layer of tomato sauce on the bottom of a shallow gratin dish, about â..." cup. Place the fennel cut sides down on top of the sauce in a tight single layer. Pour the rest of the sauce over them and spread evenly.

6. Sprinkle the fennel with the breadcrumb mixture until you have a generous crust. Drizzle with the olive oil and

bake for 30 minutes covered with foil, then 10 minutes uncovered, or until the breadcrumbs are golden.

Fish Roasted in Lemons & Tahini

This wonderful way of cooking fish comes from Lebanon. It is reminiscent of the white, nut based Mexican mole sauces. It is soothing to eat, extremely nutritious and easy to make. It's a perfect delicately tasty dish, if feeling weary due to chemo or radiotherapy. Creamy tahini with lemon is a natural complement to firm white fish. It gives it body and flavor without overwhelming its delicacy.

Ingredients
* 2 large lemons
* 1-pound thick white fish fillets
* Salt, to taste
* ½ cup tahini
* ½ cup water
* 1 tablespoon olive oil (See Chef Tips if on a Bland Diet)
* 1 large onion, halved and sliced thin (See Chef Tips if on a Bland Diet)

* parsley or cilantro, chopped

Directions

1. Preheat the oven to 425 degrees F.

2. Juice 1 of the lemons and slice the other thin.

3. Lightly oil a baking dish and place the lemon slices in the bottom of the baking dish. Rub the fish with salt and place in the center of the dish on top of just a few lemon slices, leaving some lemon slices uncovered. Roast in the oven for 20 minutes.

4. Meanwhile, in a bowl, whisk the lemon juice with tahini and water until smooth and light in color. Set aside.

5. Heat the olive oil in a wide skillet and cook the onions over medium heat until very tender and just beginning to brown, about 10 minutes. Add the onions to the tahini sauce.

6. Remove the fish from the oven and pour the tahini onion sauce over it. Return to the oven and roast for another 20-30 minutes, or until the sauce is thick and the lemon slices are well browned.

7. Discard the lemon slices under the fish, as they will be bitter. Eat warm or at room temperature, with chopped parsley or cilantro.

Spiced Beet & Tomato Soup

I came to love beets late in life. As a child, no amount of threats could make me eat the vinegary slices that we were served in the UK. Then a vegetarian friend of mine served me roasted beets. What a difference! I started to experiment. I ate borscht! This Spiced Beet & Tomato Soup started out as a curry, then one day I blended some leftovers and ended up with this gorgeous-looking, delicious spiced beet & tomato soup. The color was unbelievable. Try it with a swirl of sour cream or Greek yogurt and garnish with a pinch of cilantro

Ingredients
* 4 tablespoons grape seed or canola oil
* 1½ teaspoons whole cumin seed
* 1 large clove of garlic, thinly sliced
* 1 medium onion, coarsely chopped

* 1 teaspoon all-purpose flour

* 1/8 to ½ teaspoon ground cayenne pepper, or to taste

* 1 bunch of beets (3 to 4 roots), topped, tailed, scrubbed and cut into 6 wedges per beet

* 1½ cups chopped tomato or 1 (14-ounce) can diced tomatoes

* 1 teaspoon salt

* 1½ cups water or low-sodium vegetable stock

* Chopped cilantro to garnish (optional)

* Greek yogurt (optional)

Directions

1. Heat the oil in a medium-sized pot over medium-high heat. When the oil is hot, add the cumin seeds. Let them sizzle for a few seconds until they start to darken, then throw in the garlic. Stir-fry the garlic until it starts to turn golden. Add the onion. Stir-fry for 2 minutes until the onion softens.

2. Add the flour and cayenne. Stir and fry for a minute, taking care not to burn them. Add the beets, tomatoes, salt, and 2 cups water and bring to a simmer. Cover and turn heat to low.

3. After about 30 minutes the beets should be tender. Remove the lid and turn up the heat to medium. Cook uncovered for about 5 minutes. Use a blender to puree the soup. Adjust the seasonings and add a little water if it seems too thick -- it should have a thick, creamy consistency. Heat through over medium-low heat. Serve in bowls with a swirl of sour cream or Greek yogurt and a pinch of cilantro, if using.

CONCLUSION

Adopting a thoughtful and balanced prostate cancer diet is not just about nourishing the body, but also about empowering oneself with the tools to support overall health and well-being. By focusing on nutrient-rich foods, managing treatment side effects, and promoting a healthy lifestyle, individuals can optimize their resilience and enhance their quality of life throughout their cancer journey. Each meal becomes an opportunity to nurture both body and spirit, providing the foundation for strength, vitality, and resilience in the face of prostate cancer